UNIT

Edexcel AS | 2

Physical Education

The Critical Sports Performer

Mike Hill and Gavin Roberts

Philip Allan Updates, an imprint of Hodder Education, part of Hachette Livre UK, Market Place, Deddington, Oxfordshire OX15 0SE

Orders
Bookpoint Ltd, 130 Milton Park, Abingdon, Oxfordshire OX14 4SB
tel: 01235 827720
fax: 01235 400454
e-mail: uk.orders@bookpoint.co.uk
Lines are open 9.00 a.m.–5.00 p.m., Monday to Saturday, with a 24-hour message answering service. You can also order through the Philip Allan Updates website: www.philipallan.co.uk

ISBN 978-0-340-96677-8

First printed 2008
Impression number 5 4 3 2 1
Year 2013 2012 2011 2010 2009 2008

This guide has been written specifically to support students preparing for the Edexcel AS Physical Education Unit 2 examination. The content has been neither approved nor endorsed by Edexcel and remains the sole responsibility of the authors.

Typeset by Phoenix Photosetting, Chatham, Kent
Printed by MPG Books, Bodmin

Hachette Livre UK's policy is to use papers that are natural, renewable and recyclable products and made from wood grown in sustainable forests. The logging and manufacturing processes are expected to conform to the environmental regulations of the country of origin.

Contents

Introduction

■ ■ ■

Content Guidance

Introduction

About this guide

This unit guide is the second in a series of four, which together cover the whole of the Edexcel specification for AS and A-level Physical Education.

The AS course is assessed over two units. Unit 1 is assessed externally by means of an examination lasting 1 hour and 30 minutes, which is set and marked by Edexcel. Unit 2 involves compiling a portfolio of evidence covering four practical related tasks, which is assessed internally.

The aim of this guide is to help you prepare for Unit 2, by providing an understanding of the key concepts as well as looking at preparation strategies and assessment techniques.

The four tasks of this unit are designed to enable you to try out a range of opportunities to develop your practical experience and conduct independent research into the structure, provision and analysis of a chosen physical activity.

You will have the chance to develop your performance in two roles from a choice of three (performer, leader and official). You will need to record your performance over a period of time.

You will also need to undertake a study into the provision of sport for all three roles at a local level, followed by a study of the provision for one role at national level.

Finally you will need to produce an analysis of your practical performance in one of your roles.

This **Introduction** provides advice on how to use the guide, and an outline of the specification requirements and assessment procedures.

The **Content Guidance** section summarises the specification content of Unit 2 and gives a guide to each of the four internally assessed tasks (from Task 2.1, 'Personal performance', to Task 2.4, 'Performance analysis') that you will need to complete in order to fulfil the requirements of the unit. Although each concept is explained where necessary, you must be prepared to use other resources to improve your understanding.

How to use this guide

This guide lends itself to a number of uses throughout your Physical Education course — it is not just a *coursework* aid. Because the Content Guidance is laid out in sections that correspond to those of the specification for Unit 2, you can use it:

- to check that your notes cover the material required by the specification
- to identify strengths and weaknesses

- as a reference for what you need to cover to complete the internal tests
- during preparation of your internally assessed portfolio

The specification

In order to make the best possible start to your study of this unit, it is essential that you have access to the unit specification. This can be obtained from your teacher or directly from the awarding body, Edexcel (**www.edexcel.org.uk**).

The specification identifies everything that needs to be covered and understood. It also informs you about the assessment procedure for each part of Unit 2.

Unit description

In this unit you are assessed on four tasks:
- personal performance
- local study of sport
- national study of sport
- analysis of performance

These tasks require you to develop your practical experience in sport; to conduct independent research into the structure and provision of your sport at both local and national level; and to carry out an analysis of your chosen sport or physical activity.

You will have the chance to develop your performance in two roles from a choice of three (performer, leader and official). All three of these roles are covered in this guide.

Assessment

This unit is assessed internally. In other words, your teachers will mark your tasks and their marking will be checked by the exam board in a process called moderation. You will need to complete a portfolio of evidence that covers the four tasks — this guide takes you through each of the tasks and offers suggestions and guidance on how best to complete them. Your portfolio will need to be submitted in an electronic format, such as on a CD-ROM or DVD.

Unit 2 portfolio of evidence

You must complete all of the following four tasks:
- Task 2.1 **Personal performance** You must participate in two roles from a choice of three (performer, leader and official). This task is designed to develop your own practical performance within your chosen roles. This task is marked out of 30. You will be required to keep a log of your participation in your two roles.

- Task 2.2 **Local study** You need to undertake independent research into the provision (i.e. access, opportunities, funding, resources) for one physical activity in your local area, to cover at least one of your chosen roles. This task is marked out of 15. It will be completed as a project — there are a range of formats that you can use.
- Task 2.3 **National study** This task follows on from the previous one. In it, you need to investigate the national provision of your chosen physical activity, at elite levels, in at least one of your chosen roles. This task is marked out of 15. It will be completed as a project — there are a range of formats that you can use.
- Task 2.4 **Performance analysis** This task requires you to analyse your performance of either of the practical roles you chose in Task 2.1. This task is marked out of 30. You will need to complete the five sections and present evidence of this analysis.

One overall mark out of 90 will be submitted to the exam board at the end of the course.

Content Guidance

This section covers the content of Unit 2, which is a compulsory and internally assessed unit. Unit 2 requires you to complete four tasks or projects. In this section we will work through each task, highlighting the key areas you need to cover, and give advice and suggestions about how you can plan, research and carry out each of the tasks, and successfully complete the unit.

In Unit 2, you will have the chance to develop your performance in two roles selected from a choice of three (performer, leader and official) and you will need to record your performance over a period of time. You will then need to undertake a study into the provision of your chosen sport for all three roles at a local level, followed by a study of the provision for one role at the national level. Finally, to complete the unit, you will have to produce an analysis of your performances in one of the roles.

Task 2.1: personal performance

Introduction

You need to select two performance roles from the choice of performer, leader or official. You need to be actively involved in the two roles you choose in order to develop the quality and level of your performance. The two roles you choose can be from the same sporting activity, or you could choose different roles from two different sports.

To help you decide which roles you are best suited to, look at the following table for guidance.

Role	Description	Examples
Performer	You are an active participant in a particular sport or physical activity.	You play for your school or college team; you play, compete or train at a local sports club.
Leader	You plan and organise sporting activities. You act in a support role as a first aider or physio, and/or you carry out an analysis of the activity performed by the performer, official or leader (this is called 'activity analysis').	You coach in a school or club; you hold a sports leader's role in community sport; you help with scouts, guides or cadets.
Official	You officiate in a sport at a level appropriate to your qualifications and experience.	You referee lower school matches; you act as scorer/timekeeper/judge for local club teams; you help organise local TOP Link festivals.

Tip If you are still not sure which two roles to choose, think about which you can talk most about. In all the tasks for Unit 2, you will need to discuss and research a great deal of information.

Pathway 1: the performer

Key points

You are required to undertake one practical performance in a sporting activity and to perform in both structured practices and competition.

You need to work on developing your performance over a period of at least 8 weeks.

How will you be assessed?

As a practical performer, you are required to participate in your chosen sport for a minimum of 8 weeks, taking part in a combination of structured practices and competitive performances, tournaments or events. While being assessed, you must demonstrate to the examiner your ability to perform in both structured practices and competitive situations. In addition, you are required to produce evidence of full active participation in a minimum of three formal organised performances appropriate to your personal level.

> **Tip** Before you start your practical unit, think about the strengths and weaknesses of your current performance. What are the key areas you need to work on?

> **Key terms**
>
> **Structured practices** — these are opportunities where individuals or groups engage in an organised performance environment in order to enhance and refine their own personal performance. In this context the practices should be arranged in a way that enables the performer to show his or her optimum level of ability while still demonstrating the full range of skills required.
>
> **Organised performances** — these are situations where individuals or teams/groups are able to produce a planned response to a scenario or set of circumstances. This may include a competitive match (individual or team), a gymnastics or dance routine, or a timed expedition.

The examiner will look at three areas:
- **Your ability to perform the skills required in the sport of your choice.** When assessing you in this area, the examiner will consider:
  - the range of skills that you can perform
  - the level at which you perform them
  - the effectiveness of your execution of the skills
  - the consistency of your performance of the skills
- **Your ability to apply the skills in a variety of situations.** Consideration will be given to:
  - your understanding of the correct language and terminology
  - your ability to select the appropriate skill at the correct time
  - your ability to adapt the skills appropriately to the environment

- **Your ability to analyse and adapt performance in a competitive situation to achieve success.** Here the examiner will be looking at:
  - the effect of the pressure of competition on your skill level
  - your generic ability to influence the activity
  - your ability to influence the activity specifically when attacking and defending
  - your ability to adapt your own performance in relation to that of your opponents
  - your ability to apply different tactics and strategies to maximise your success and minimise your opponents' chances of succeeding
  - the number of unforced errors that you make and your ability to force your opponent into such errors

Grading the performance

The examiner will grade you within one of five bands. The bands are as follows:

- Band 1: 1–3 marks
- Band 2: 4–6 marks
- Band 3: 7–9 marks
- Band 4: 10–12 marks
- Band 5: 13–15 marks

You need to present evidence of full active participation in a minimum of three formal organised performances at a level appropriate to your age group and ability.

Observation and correction

You need to be able to pick out faults in both your own performance and that of others. What is going wrong? Why are you not being successful?

Having identified a problem, the next step is to decide what to do about it. Before you can do this you need to have a sound knowledge of the skills and tactics required for each activity. Coaching qualifications and courses will help, but your PE lessons should give you enough information and experience to do some basic observation and correction.

The best way to observe a performance

Filming a performer has the advantage of allowing you to stop, repeat and slow down the performance. This makes it much easier to identify faults. However, it is not always practical to use video, especially in sports such as swimming. So you need to be able to carry out live observation.

The first part of live observation and correction is to have in your mind a clear picture of what you should be seeing, that is, a perfect or near-perfect attempt. Demonstrations or books can give you this perfect model. You then need to judge the performance you are watching against this mental model. You can make your analysis easier by dividing the skill or the performer's body into smaller parts and concentrating on these one at a time.

For example, if you are looking at a long-jumper, you could divide up the activity as follows:

Skill	Body part
Run-up	Legs
Take-off	Arms
Flight	Head
Landing	Torso

Splitting the skill up into smaller parts or subroutines should make it easier to observe, identify faults and offer suggestions for correction. However, this may mean your performer repeating the activity many times. It helps to have a thorough knowledge of the relevant coaching points.

How will I score marks on this assignment?

Your centre assessor and the external examiner will look at the evidence of your performance and then use a grid similar to the one below to give your performance a mark out of 15. You can use this grid as a checklist for your own performance. Although most of the content reads the same, there are key words to look for in each phrase — we have put these in bold to make them easier for you to identify.

Band	Description
Band 5 13–15 marks	The performer has produced a **very high level** of very consistent performances in both the short-term preparation and the long-term training for the appropriate competitive environments of his/her selected sports activity.
	The performer, during the length of the assessment period, has been able to perform at **first level elite representation**, and probably beyond, with the basis of this performance being centred on a high standard of the appropriate physiological, technical, tactical and psychological aspects related to his/her sports activity.
	In competition, the performer has been able to produce **dominant performances** in a variety of competitive formats and is able to respond to, and use, the pressure of expectation to achieve successes at his/her level of performance/participation.
Band 4 10–12 marks	The performer has produced a **high level** of consistent performances in both the short-term preparation and the long-term training for the appropriate competitive environments of his/her selected sports activity.
	The performer, during the length of the assessment period, has been able to perform in **some form of representative sport** at school/college or club level, while generally being a 'first choice', with the basis of this performance being centred on a very good standard of the appropriate physiological, technical, tactical and psychological aspects related to his/her sports activity.

continued

Band	Description
	In competition, the performer has been able to produce **consistent performances** in a variety of competitive formats and is able to cope with the pressure of expectation to achieve successes at his/her level of performance/participation.
Band 3 7–9 marks	The performer has produced a **good level** of consistent performances in both the short-term preparation and the long-term training for the appropriate competitive environments of his/her selected sports activity.
	The performer, during the length of the assessment period, has been able to perform in **some form of representative sport** at school/college or club level, while not always being a 'first choice', with the basis of this performance being centred on a good standard of the appropriate physiological, technical, tactical and psychological aspects related to his/her sports activity.
	In competition, the performer has been able to produce **reasonably consistent performances** in a variety of competitive formats and is invariably able to cope with the pressure of expectation to achieve successes at his/her level of performance/participation.
Band 2 4–6 marks	The performer has produced a **rudimentary level** of inconsistent performances in both the short-term preparation and the long-term training for the appropriate competitive environments of his/her selected sports activity.
	The performer, during the length of the assessment period, has been able to perform in **some form of representative sport** at school/college or club level, while not always being a 'first choice', with the basis of this performance being centred on an average but limited standard of the appropriate physiological, technical, tactical and psychological aspects related to his/her sports activity.
	In competition, the performer has been able produce **reasonably consistent performances** in a variety of competitive formats and is invariably able to cope with the pressure of expectation to achieve successes at his/her level of performance/participation.
Band 1 1–3 marks	The performer has produced a performance **in line with a beginner** in both the short-term preparation and the long-term training for the appropriate competitive environments of his/her selected sports activity.
	The performer, during the length of the assessment period, has **rarely been able to perform in some form of representative sport** at school/college or club level, with the basis of this performance being centred on a poor standard of the appropriate physiological, technical, tactical and psychological aspects related to his/her sports activity.
	If involved in competition, the performer has been able to produce **very inconsistent performances** in a variety of competitive formats and is invariably unable to cope with the pressure of expectation to achieve successes at his/her level of performance/participation.

Pathway 2: the leader in sport

Key points

You need to present evidence of your involvement as a leader in a sporting context. This role could include undertaking the responsibility for training and the competitive preparation of an individual or team (working as a coach) or acting as part of a medical team or in other roles such as a sports psychologist or tournament organiser.

You may be able to provide evidence of your preparation for such a role through either undertaking recognised leadership courses or national governing body awards.

How will you be assessed?

You need to provide evidence of your experience of, and learning in, a leadership role in a particular physical activity.

You can show proof of your preparation for such a leadership role through the successful completion of recognised leadership and/or coaching courses.

Coaching and leadership in sport and physical recreation

In the UK:
- 1.2 million individuals regularly coach sport (1 in 50 of the UK population).
- Six million sports volunteers are actively involved in helping out with sporting events or activities.
- The large majority of coaching in the UK is carried out by non-qualified, unpaid, part-time volunteers.

Improving your skills as a leader or coach
- Know your sport: key areas are tactics, skills and training methods that can be used to improve performance.
- Keep learning: read, take courses, watch others lead and coach.
- Motivate your performers: make all your sessions fun but challenging.
- Understand the needs of your performers: identify their strengths and weaknesses and work out which style of leadership they respond to best.
- Communicate effectively: explain clearly what you mean; use demonstrations as much as possible and listen to your performers.
- Lead by example: be a role model in terms of behaviour, dress and attitude.

Sports leaders awards

These are overseen by Sports Leaders UK. They are aimed primarily at school and college students. There is a progressive suite of awards.

Level 1 award in sports leadership
This is an award for those aged over 14. It gives an insight into leadership and helps

develop generic leadership skills. It is a practical course, examined through observation rather than written tests.

Award in dance leadership

This qualification is for those aged over 14. It uses the medium of dance to help develop leadership skills. The course does not require candidates to be expert dancers. Candidates work to complete a log book and are required to lead a dance activity that they have planned and organised.

Level 2 award in community sports leadership

This award is for candidates aged over 16. It develops the skills and knowledge required to plan and deliver safe sporting and recreational sessions. The award includes eight practical units and candidates complete a log book as well as undertaking at least 10 hours of leading community sport.

Level 2 award in basic expedition leadership

This award is aimed at people aged over 17 who are interested in outdoor sports and activities. The course develops the skills and experience to organise safe outdoor expeditions and overnight camps. Successful completion of the course requires the compilation of a log book and 30 hours of leadership experience under supervision.

Level 3 award in higher sports leadership

Candidates must be aged 18 or over on completion of the course and must have previously completed the Level 2 award. The award contains both practical and written work, though the emphasis is on practical application. Candidates must also undertake a minimum of 30 hours of leadership in community sport.

Sports-specific coaching awards

Most national governing bodies (NGBs) run their own portfolios of coaching and leadership awards. Candidates who achieve one of these qualifications can be sure that they have received training in the best coaching techniques and the latest thinking in sport. A further benefit of an NGB coaching award is that it gives the holder liability insurance, which covers against accidents that could happen when coaching (this usually only applies to Level 1 awards and above).

Most NGB coaching qualifications are based on the following framework:

Level	Title	Description
Foundation	Beginner or leader's award	Usually aimed at young people or those who want to get involved in coaching. Usually consists of around 9 hours of training.
1	Coaching assistant	For coaches aged 16+ who will be introducing sport to young people or inexperienced adults in a safe and planned manner. Usually consists of around 16 hours of training.

Level	Title	Description
2	Coach	For those aged 17+ who have already achieved Level 1. Level 2 courses require the completion of a coaching log book in which candidates record sessions that they have planned and delivered. Duration of the courses is normally 60–90 hours.
3	Club coach/senior coach	Aimed at those aged 18+ who already have at least 30 hours of coaching experience. The course normally requires the completion of a log book and contains practical assessment of candidates' coaching skills and both oral and written examinations.
4	Master/elite coach	For appointed coaches of elite teams and performers. The courses require the completion of a log book and practical assessment, and can take up to 18 months to complete.

Some sports have a Level 5 award aimed at national team coaches.

You should be aware that different qualifications mean different things in different sports. Not all coaching qualifications allow you to coach alone or to lead a session. Some (often those below Level 2) only allow an individual to work under the guidance of a more qualified coach.

There are likely to be changes in the scope of NGB coaching qualifications as NGBs move towards adopting the standards laid down by the new UK Coaching Certificate. For these reasons, we recommend that you contact your relevant NGB or County Sports Association to check the types and levels of courses that are available in your sport.

The role of Sports Coach UK

Sports Coach UK is a charitable organisation and is the lead agency for the development of the UK coaching system. Its aim is to create a world-class coaching system in the UK. Most of the organisation's work involves supporting and encouraging coaches. This is done through a network of 45 coaching development officers who work closely with their county sports partnerships to develop and support continuous professional development for coaches.

The coaching development officers run regional workshops, which offer a series of qualifications that you might find useful and which should help you develop as a coach or leader. These workshops fall into two categories: coaching essentials and developing your coaching.

Coaching essentials

This is a series of seven linked workshops designed for people interested in, or with limited experience of, coaching, who want to know more about what good, safe and effective coaching is.

Developing your coaching

This consists of a series of 22 linked workshops covering a range of topics from equity through to injury prevention and management. These workshops are for coaches who want to develop their coaching skills and knowledge further to provide high-quality coaching sessions.

For more information on the work of Sports Coach UK or to check what is happening in your region, follow the links at **www.sportscoachuk.org**.

UK Coaching Certificate (UKCC)

The UKCC, managed and developed by Sports Coach UK, was set up in order to respond to the UK government's plans for sport. The certificate aims to:
- advance coaching education programmes and practices
- support the development of coaching as a profession

The qualification has five levels that create a progressive pathway for coaches to follow. These five levels are listed in the table.

Level	What the coach will be qualified to do	Experience required
5	Generate, direct and manage cutting-edge coaching programmes	Expert
4	Design and implement long-term and specialist coaching programmes	
3	Plan, implement and analyse annual coaching programmes	
2	Prepare, deliver and review coaching sessions	
1	Assist a more qualified coach	Beginner

Other sports leadership qualifications and workshops

Running Sports is Sport England's education and training programme for volunteers, created in 1997. The service offers online tips, case studies and tools, as well as workshops through the county sports partnerships. More information is available at **www.runningsports.org**.

Why should I do a coaching or leadership qualification?

There are a number of excellent reasons for doing a coaching/leadership course. Gaining such a qualification will help you to:
- improve your knowledge on how to plan a safe and enjoyable coaching or leadership session
- gain new and up-to-date ideas and techniques

- find out about new legislation in your sport
- gain insurance cover from your sport's governing body

Help

Local authority sports development services offer advice and information on gaining qualifications in sport and may also run a range of courses themselves.

Child protection and the sports leader

In response to the government's Every Child Matters strategy, all clubs and voluntary organisations have statutory duties and responsibilities in relation to safeguarding and protecting children and young people. All governing bodies in sport now appoint a lead child protection officer and have developed sports-specific guidelines that you need to be aware of before leading, teaching or coaching children.

> **Key term**
>
> **Every Child Matters strategy** — this strategy has identified the following key outcomes for all children and young people:
> - Be healthy
> - Stay safe
> - Enjoy and achieve
> - Make a positive contribution
> - Achieve economic wellbeing

Child protection in practice

As a sports leader, there are a number of child protection guidelines you should follow:
- Always work in an 'open' environment, avoiding situations where you are alone with young people or where you cannot be observed.
- Treat all your charges equally and with respect and dignity.
- Make sporting activity fun and enjoyable, and promote fair play in competition.
- Be an excellent role model — for example, never swear, smoke or drink alcohol in the company of young people.
- Give enthusiastic and constructive feedback rather than negative criticism.

The duty of the sports club, team or facility

All clubs and organisations have to recognise that everyone has the potential to abuse children in some way. In light of this, they have to take reasonable steps to ensure that unsuitable people are prevented from working with children within their facilities.

As a result, when taking up a position with a sports club or organisation you may be asked to provide some or all of the following:
- an application form requiring you to disclose any information regarding criminal activity
- a consent form that allows the club or organisation to seek a Criminal Records Bureau (CRB) check (see below)
- evidence of identity, such as a copy of your passport or driving licence

- the names and contact details of referees who can report on your suitability or previous work with children and young people

  Tip For more information on child protection and how it affects your role as a sports leader, check out the Child Protection in Sport Unit website at **www.thecpsu.org.uk.**

Criminal Records Bureau (CRB) checks

As a sports leader working in community sport, you may be asked to submit to a CRB check. The Criminal Records Bureau can check police records and records held by the government departments of Health and Children, Schools and Families. Organisations such as sports clubs and schools use the service when appointing teachers, as well as coaches, instructors and sports leaders. There are two types of CRB check: standard disclosure or enhanced disclosure. Both require payment of a fee but are free of charge to volunteers.

In most cases relating to sport, a **standard disclosure** is undertaken. A standard disclosure shows any current or past convictions, cautions, reprimands and warnings that are held about a person on the police national computer. If your coaching and leadership involves contact with children, the Protection of Children Act list is also checked. (This is information held under Section 142 of the Education Act of 2002 — it was formally known as List 99.)

An **enhanced disclosure** is asked for when people are appointed full time into jobs where they will be in sole charge of children and young people, such as a PE teacher or sports development officer. The enhanced disclosure contains the same informa- tion as the standard disclosure but also includes a search of information held by local police forces as well as the national database.

How will I score marks on this assignment?

Your centre assessor and the external examiner will look at the evidence of your performance and then use a grid similar to the one below to give your performance a mark out of 15. You can use this grid as a checklist for your own performance. Although most of the content reads the same, there are key words to look for in each phrase — we have put these in bold to make them easier for you to identify.

Band	Description
Band 5 13–15 marks	The leader has produced a **very high level** of performance in leading a group, team or individual in one sporting context during the length of the assessment period.
	The leader has demonstrated, through a **high level** of applied knowledge and understanding, how to work alongside others in order to progress performances in a sports environment appropriate to the leader's ability and specific role.
	continued

Band	Description
	The learner is **fully able** to recognise and act upon the strengths and weaknesses of the group, team or individual, and is highly proficient in communicating, displays **extensive** organisational abilities and motivational skills, while working at, or aspiring to work at, an elite level at or close to his/her own age group.
Band 4 10–12 marks	The leader has produced a **high level** of performance in leading a group, team or individual in one sporting context during the length of the assessment period. The leader has demonstrated, through an **informed level** of applied knowledge and understanding, how to work alongside others in order to progress performances in a sports environment appropriate to the leader's ability and specific role. The leader is **able** to recognise and act upon the strengths and weaknesses of the group, team or individual, and is proficient in communicating, displays **very good** organisational abilities and motivational skills, while aspiring to work at an elite level out of his/her own age group.
Band 3 7–9 marks	The leader has produced a **good level** of performance in leading a group, team or individual in one sporting context during the length of the assessment period. The leader has demonstrated, through a **sound level** of applied knowledge and understanding, how to work alongside others in order to progress performances in a sports environment appropriate to the leader's ability and specific role. The leader is **normally able** to recognise and act upon the strengths and weaknesses of the group, team or individual, is developing his/her communication skills and displays **good** organisational abilities and motivational skills. The leader is working at a level below his/her own age group, which may not involve elite performers.
Band 2 4–6 marks	The leader has produced a **rudimentary level** of performance in leading a group, team or individual in one sporting context during the length of the assessment period. The leader has demonstrated, through an **emerging level** of applied knowledge and understanding, how to work alongside others in order to progress performances in a sports environment appropriate to the leader's ability and specific role. The leader is **sometimes able** to recognise and act upon the strengths and weaknesses of the group, team or individual, and has limited communication skills and organisational abilities, while demonstrating few motivational skills. The leader is only able to work at a level below his/her own age group, which will probably not involve elite performers.
Band 1 1–3 marks	The leader has produced a performance in line with a **beginner** in leading a group, team or individual in one sporting context during the length of the assessment period. *continued*

Band	Description
	The leader has demonstrated, through a **basic level** of applied knowledge and understanding, how to work alongside others in order to progress performances in a sports environment appropriate to the leader's ability and specific role.
	The leader is **rarely able** to recognise and act upon the strengths and weaknesses of the group, team or individual, and has very limited communication skills and organisational abilities, while demonstrating minimal motivational skills. The leader is only able to work at a level much below his/her own age group, which will not involve elite performers.

Self-evaluation checklist for leaders

Item required	Tick when completed
Appearance • I looked smart and confident before, during and after my session.	
Planning • I had planned my session thoroughly. • I had included contingency plans in case something had to be changed in my plan.	
Preparation • I had time to arrange equipment and the session before the participants arrived. • All the equipment and kit I needed was available.	
Communication • I was not distracted by anything or anyone during the session. • My instructions were clear and concise. • My coaching points were short and to the point. • The performers understood my instructions and were able to undertake all tasks.	
Appropriateness of sessions • Players were able to complete the task and drills I set them. • The conditioned games and activities highlighted the skills required. • There was an appropriate warm-up and cool-down.	
Control and authority • I felt I had the respect of the players and that they responded well to my actions. • I responded to the needs of the players and I adapted drills and tasks to suit their abilities.	

Pathway 3: the sports official

Key points

If you choose the role of an official, you will need to provide evidence of your preparation for active participation in a chosen physical activity in this capacity. One excellent way of proving this is to study for a national governing body (NGB) award or other officiating qualification to prove your proficiency further.

How will you be assessed?

You need to officiate (and be recorded) in at least three competitive situations or in a single tournament appropriate to your level of ability.

In this guide, we concentrate on the following official roles: umpires, line judges, time keepers, scorers, linesmen, referees, fourth officials, video referees and judges. Your sport may have other examples of officials, so check with your tutor or teacher to see if you can use these roles in your preparation for the unit.

The role of an official in sport

An official in sport is defined as any person who controls the actual play of a sports competition by applying the rules and laws of that specific sport. Officials need to make judgements on rule infringement, performance, scores and time allocations. They play a central role in ensuring that everyone involved — performers and coaches — observes the spirit of the game.

Officials have been involved in sport for thousands of years. We know that at the ancient Olympics in Greece, special officials called Hellanodikai were appointed to oversee the running of the games and settle any disputes between performers. So important was their role, they were required to live for 10 months in seclusion prior to the games to help them prepare and to be away from coaches and spectators who might try to influence their decisions during the games. The Hellanodikais' decisions were final, and athletes and their coaches faced harsh punishments if they broke any of the Olympian rules.

The official's role in sport came of age at the end of the nineteenth century, when the majority of modern sports went through a period referred to as rationalisation — governing bodies were formed, and standardised sets of rules were created and distributed. From then on, it became the role of the officials to ensure that these rules were adhered to.

Key characteristics of a sports official

The role is a demanding one. Officials must have a thorough understanding of the game and be able to communicate effectively with players, coaches and spectators. They need to keep a calm head in what can become very tense situations, especially in sports finals where one decision could mean the difference between winning and losing.

It is the duty of the officials to interpret and apply the rules, and they have the right to ignore protests.

What do officials in sport do?

There are a number of key roles that officials play. These roles may not all apply to your selected sport, so you need to choose the most appropriate one to use in your assignment.

- **Arbiter** — the person who makes the final decision
- **Judge** — someone who makes a decision after considering a range of factors
- **Communicator** — an official needs to use both verbal and non-verbal communication methods that everyone involved in the game understands
- **Timekeeper** — the person who ensures the game is played within the official time limits
- **Score keeper** — someone who keeps a formal record of the score as the game progresses (an important role)
- **Safety officer** — someone who ensures that everyone involved in the game participates in a safe and secure way

When working with younger players, the official's role changes slightly. As well as applying the rules, he/she needs to act as a role model and educator, showing the principles of fair and unbiased decision-making, as well as explaining decisions and how the rules of the game work.

If your role is as an assistant referee or umpire, you will have a number of other roles and responsibilities. Your job in this case is to help the referee make decisions and to act as an extra pair of eyes. In sports such as football and rugby, for example, it is usual for each assistant to be responsible for a specific part or half of the pitch and to make decisions regarding the boundaries of play. They also rule on offside. Assistant referees assist with substitutions, signalling to the referee that a team wishes to make a substitution, and may also check the new player's kit and appearance before he/she enters the game. It should be noted, though, that in general an assistant only signals to the referee and does not make the actual decisions.

Remember:

- The referee makes the final decision.
- Make your signals clear and decisive.
- Keep up with play — in most sports there is a 'line of sight' across the pitch, where you need to be.
- Assistant referees should be silent during the game. They may not coach or direct the players in any way.

Child protection and the sports official

In response to the government's Every Child Matters strategy, all clubs and voluntary organisations have statutory duties and responsibilities in relation to safeguarding and protecting children and young people. All governing bodies in sport now appoint a lead child protection officer and have developed sports-specific guidelines that you need to be aware of before working with children or young people in your role as a sports official.

Key term

Every Child Matters strategy — this strategy has identified the following key outcomes for all children and young people:
- Be healthy
- Stay safe
- Enjoy and achieve
- Make a positive contribution
- Achieve economic wellbeing

Child protection in practice

As a sports official, there are a number of child protection guidelines you should follow:
- Always work in an 'open' environment, avoiding situations where you are alone with young people or where you cannot be observed.
- Treat all your charges equally and with respect and dignity.
- Make sporting activity fun and enjoyable, and promote fair play in competition.
- Be an excellent role model — for example, never swear, smoke or drink alcohol in the company of young people.
- Give enthusiastic and constructive feedback rather than negative criticism.

Child protection and the recruitment and training of staff and volunteers

All clubs and organisations have to recognise that everyone has the potential to abuse children in some way. In light of this, they have to take reasonable steps to ensure that unsuitable people are prevented from working with children within their facilities.

As a result, when taking up a position with a sports club or organisation you may be asked to provide some or all of the following:
- an application form requiring you to disclose any information regarding criminal activity
- a consent form that allows the club or organisation to seek a Criminal Records Bureau (CRB) check (see below)
- evidence of identity, such as a copy of your passport or driving licence
- the names and contact details of referees who can report on your suitability or previous work with children and young people

Tip For more information on child protection and how it affects your role as a sports official, check out the Child Protection in Sport Unit website at **www.thecpsu.org.uk.**

Criminal Records Bureau checks (CRB)

As a sports official working in community sport, you may be asked to submit to a CRB check. The Criminal Records Bureau can check police records and records held by the government departments of Health and Children, Schools and Families.

Organisations such as sports clubs and schools use the service when appointing teachers, as well as coaches, instructors and sports leaders. There are two types of CRB check: standard disclosure or enhanced disclosure. Both require payment of a fee but are free of charge to volunteers.

In most cases relating to sport, a **standard disclosure** is undertaken. A standard disclosure shows any current or past convictions, cautions, reprimands and warnings that are held about a person on the police national computer. If your coaching and leadership involves contact with children, the Protection of Children Act list is also checked. (This is information held under Section 142 of the Education Act of 2002 — it was formerly known as List 99.)

An **enhanced disclosure** is asked for when people are appointed full time into jobs where they will be in sole charge of children and young people, such as a PE teacher or sports development officer. The enhanced disclosure contains the same informa-tion as the standard disclosure but also includes a search of information held by local police forces as well as the national database.

What makes a good official?

Being a good official requires a delicate balance. The best officials blend into the background of the game and yet are able at the same time to show their presence and be authoritative. The basic requirements for good officiating are:

- being firm and fair without officiousness or arrogance
- being impartial
- applying the rules and/or score without pressure from players, coaches or fans
- gaining the respect of players, coaches and spectators
- being confident

The managers and coaches of teams that have just narrowly lost a game often blame their disappointment on a decision made by the official. However, it is worth remembering that losing a match usually has more to do with mistakes committed by players and coaches during the game than it does with one mistake by the referee. The higher up the performance pyramid you go, the more coaches and players have invested in the outcome of their games (often linked to financial rewards) and the less tolerant they become of the rules, each other and especially the decisions of the officials.

The role of the official therefore becomes more and more difficult and pressured, depending on the importance of the match or game. So it is essential to reflect thoroughly on the qualities of a good official, as listed above.

Does the official need to have played the game?

This is a topic for heated debate in sport, especially at the elite level. Being able to apply the rules and interpret why or how a player took a certain action, some would argue, can only be truly understood by those who have played the game at some level. Experience gained as a performer, they surmise, enables an official to draw on personal experience when making a tough call. However, it can also be argued that thinking like a player does not always mean that the rules are stringently applied. Individuals who have little or no previous competitive experience but are dedicated students of their sport and its rules can and do develop into effective game officials. The key point is that the officials must gain the respect and confidence of the performers. In some sports, being an ex-player may help foster such respect; in others it may have little value.

Understanding the rules

Understanding the rules of the game is an essential starting point for all sports officials. However, remember that rules do change, so you need constantly to review those for your particular sport. Making effective calls and decisions is also about the mechanics of officiating, so you need to learn the proper positions for the different officials' roles and practise them until positioning becomes second nature. Making the correct signals lets everybody know what decision you have come to and helps stamp your authority on the game. The timing of decisions is another skill you need to master; it can sometimes be just as valuable to allow play to continue as to call a halt for every tiny infringement, for instance.

Physical fitness

Just as performers need to be fit for their sport, so too do officials. After all, they need to be able to keep up with players and still have the mental stamina to make the call. Most officials undergo pre-season fitness training to help them prepare for the physical demands of the job, as well as continuing with regular training sessions to keep in shape throughout the season itself.

Tip Both the FA and the Referees' Association websites give details of a range of training programmes for all levels of referees and assistant referees. You can look them up at **www.thefa.com** and **www.footballreferee.org**.

Improving your performance as an official

Most sports governing bodies have well-structured development pathways for referees and officials. It would be a good idea to work out where you are on this pathway at present and which level to aim for in terms of progression. In order to move up a level, it is usually necessary to undertake further training and some form of assessment.

Improving fitness is also a requirement for the higher levels of officiating, so it would be useful to include an assessment of your current fitness as well as suggestions for both targets and training plans that would enable you to meet the increased fitness demands.

Tip Key areas that you could consider when planning how to improve your performance as an official could include:
- practice
- training

- further qualifications
- self-analysis
- buddy systems (working with another official or more so that you can share advice and experiences)

There is a wide range of methods and programmes, examples of which are listed below, that you could consider when drawing up your development plan as a sports official. The value of these depends on both your official role and the specific sport.

- **Referees courses and retraining** — most governing bodies offer a pathway of progressive qualifications. You will find that the higher the level of qualification, the longer and more demanding the courses will be.
- **Websites** — there are a number of websites dedicated to officials in sport, which may offer ideas and techniques that you could apply. Examples include **www.naso.org**, **www.referee.com** and **www.sportsofficialsuk.com**.
- **Special clinics** — local and regional associations often put on clinics and workshops where officials can share ideas and discuss rules and regulations. Top-level officials are frequently invited to lead the sessions. Try to find out if your sport has local forums for sports officials.
- **Publications** — most governing bodies produce handbooks and guidelines for officials, which may be available as PDF downloads on websites. For more popular sports, such as football and tennis, there are also independent texts and handbooks, such as *An Introduction to Sports Officiating* by David Pegg (Coachwise Ltd, 2005), *Calling the Play: A Beginner's Guide to Amateur Sports Officiating* by Edward Dolan (Atheneum, 1981) and *Modern Sports Officiating: A Practical Guide* by Richard Clegg and William Thompson (Brown, 1989). As a minimum, make sure you have up-to-date copies of the sports rules and regulations.
- **Officiating at local tournaments** — although it is hard work, having to referee a lot of short games played close together provides invaluable experience. It also creates the opportunity to watch and meet other officials.
- **Games** — refereeing or watching as many games as you can is the best way to develop knowledge and technique. Try to step up to officiate in adult or more senior games.
- **Assessors** — formal assessments are part of almost any governing body development pathway. They give valuable feedback and often contain specific areas for improvement. Assessors can be sounding boards too, and valuable for bouncing ideas and thoughts off.
- **Friends, colleagues, associates, players, coaches, mentors, administrators** — talk to them. Listen to what they say. Discount some of it, where obviously biased, but listen all the same. Get inputs and insights. Shared information is a better builder of knowledge than uncertain solitary wonderings. Stockpile everything you learn.

How to officiate effectively in a selected sport

As an official in a sport, your key aim is to allow the game to progress smoothly and within the rules. This will be achieved by you being in the correct position to see the play, reacting immediately to rule infractions, and making all the players aware of your decisions through both verbal and non-verbal communication.

It may be worth considering working out a plan of action for the games you have to officiate, as outlined below.

Before play starts

- Arrive at least 30 minutes early.
- Warm up properly.
- Introduce yourself to players and coaches. This may be a good time to talk through any key rules and regulations, especially if there have been any recent updates by governing bodies. It is also usual to agree on a channel of communication on the field (normally through the captains).
- Don't oversell yourself — be polite and friendly, but remember that coaches and players will expect you to maintain a distance.
- Look over the playing area and identify any potential problems.

During the game

- Don't overanticipate — it is better to be a split second late rather than blow early and rule incorrectly.
- Don't rush your signals, as these are often missed by the players. Rushing is often caused by being overanxious, so try to stay as calm as you can.
- Enforce all rules, especially early in the game. You will want the game to flow and may consider overlooking minor infringements, but doing this too early can lead to frustration among the players and tempt them to take the law into their own hands.
- Keep communicating with players and your fellow officials.
- Keep checking your positioning and follow the flow of the game. Don't forget to use any breaks in play to enable you to move to a better position.
- Don't overreact to complaints. Be calm and firm and penalise any dissent.

After the game

- If you get the chance, discuss the game with other officials present, asking for advice or suggestions they might have about your performance.
- Have a small notebook handy, where you can note down key points from the game. This will make it easier to write up your assignment later. What did you feel were your strengths and areas for improvement? Have you learned any new rules or techniques for the game? Do you have any queries about the rules and regulations that you will need to look up or ask about?

Self-evaluation checklist for officials

Appearance

- Did I look smart and confident before, during and after the game I officiated?
- Was I distracted by anything or anyone during the game?

Signals
- Did I use the whistle effectively and with confidence?
- Did I always use signals to back up the decisions I gave?

Stopping play
- Were there any incidents of time-wasting and did I deal with them effectively?
- Was I effective in getting the game restarted after stoppages?

Advantage
- Did I make it clear to the players I was allowing advantage?
- Did I speak to offenders after advantage had been played?
- If no advantage accrued, did I stop the game and penalise the original offence?

Cooperation with other officials
- Did I seek advice from the other officials?
- How well did I communicate with the other officials?

Offences
- Did I identify and take control of dangerous play?

Positioning
- Did I anticipate play well and feel I was always in the best position to make a decision?
- Did my positioning during set plays allow me a clear view of all concerned players?
- Did I manage to keep a distance from the immediate location of play that allowed me an overall view of the pitch and players?
- Did I use stoppages effectively to enable me to move into the best position for the next phase of play?

Control and authority
- Did I feel I had the respect of the players and that they responded well to my actions?
- Did I deal calmly but firmly with any dissent?
- Did I hesitate in making any of my decisions?

How will I score marks on this assignment?

Your centre assessor and the external examiner will look at the evidence of your performance and then use a grid similar to the one below to give your performance a mark out of 15. You can use this grid as a checklist for your own performance. Although most of the content reads the same, there are key words to look for in each phrase — we have put these in bold to make them easier for you to identify.

Band	Description
Band 5 13–15 marks	The official has been able to produce a **very high standard** of officiating at an appropriate performance level in one selected sports activity during the length of the assessment period. *continued*

Band	Description
	The official demonstrates an **extensive** knowledge and understanding of the rules/laws of the selected sports activity and can always impose authority when required to ensure that the performance is successful.
	The official has **excellent** communication, positioning and signalling skills as appropriate to the level of competition and his/her experience and/or recognised NGB qualification(s).
	The official **always** carries out his/her responsibilities with the required uniform, equipment and pre-officiating protocols, as required to meet the highest standards.
	The official has a **full awareness** of the performance demands required of the participant(s).
Band 4 10–12 marks	The official has been able to produce a **high standard** of officiating at an appropriate performance level in one selected sports activity during the length of the assessment period.
	The official demonstrates a **proficient** knowledge and understanding of the rules/laws of the selected sports activity and can, on most occasions, impose authority when required to ensure that the performance is successful.
	The official has **very good** communication, positioning and signalling skills as appropriate to the level of competition and his/her experience and/or recognised NGB qualification(s).
	The official can **usually** be relied upon to carry out his/her responsibilities with the required uniform, equipment and pre-officiating protocols, as required to meet very good standards.
	The official has **an awareness** of the performance demands required of the sports participant(s).
Band 3 7–9 marks	The official has been able to produce a **good standard** of officiating at an appropriate performance level in one selected sports activity during the length of the assessment period.
	The official demonstrates a **sound** knowledge and understanding of the rules/laws of the selected sports activity and can usually, but not always, impose authority when required to ensure that the performance is successful.
	The official has **good** communication, positioning and signalling skills as appropriate to the level of competition and his/her experience, but may not hold recognised NGB qualification(s).
	The official can **generally** be relied upon to carry out his/her responsibilities with the required uniform, equipment and pre-officiating protocols, as required to meet reasonable standards.
	The official has a **limited awareness** of the performance demands required of the sports participant(s).

Band	Description
Band 2 4–6 marks	The official has been able to produce a **rudimentary standard** of officiating at an appropriate performance level in one selected sports activity during the length of the assessment period. The official demonstrates an **emerging** knowledge and understanding of the rules/laws of the selected sports activity and can only occasionally impose authority when required to ensure that the performance is successful. The official has **limited** communication, positioning and signalling skills as appropriate to the level of competition and his/her experience, but will probably not hold recognised NGB qualification(s). The official can **rarely** be relied upon to carry out his/her responsibilities with the required uniform, equipment and pre-officiating protocols, as required to meet reasonable standards. The official has a **limited awareness** of the performance demands required of the sports participant(s).
Band 1 1–3 marks	The official has produced a performance in line with a **beginner** officiating at an appropriate performance level in one selected sports activity during the length of the assessment period. The official demonstrates a **very limited** knowledge and understanding of the rules/laws of the selected sports activity and can rarely impose authority when required to ensure that the performance is successful. The student has **poor** communication, positioning and signalling skills as appropriate to the level of competition and his/her experience, and will have no recognised NGB qualification(s). The official can **very rarely** be relied upon to carry out his/her responsibilities with the required uniform, equipment and pre-officiating protocols, as required to meet reasonable standards. The official has a **scant awareness** of the performance demands required of the sports participant(s).

Task 2.2: local study

Key points

You need to research and present a study of the local provision and opportunities for participation in one chosen physical activity. Your study should:

- include grass roots and the first level of elite selection
- reflect the school, college, club and area provisions in terms of facilities, organisations, competitions available and the opportunity for development
- cover the three roles of performer, leader and official

How will you be assessed?

There is no set format for Task 2.2, so you can present your work in a range of ways. You should choose a style that you are familiar with or that you think will best present the information you discover on sport in your local area.

Your presentation must be limited to 1,000 words if you are writing in continuous prose. Teacher assessors and moderators will discontinue marking once the prescribed word limit is reached.

Some examples of the type of format you could choose include:
- a brochure that illustrates your physical activity in the local area
- a PowerPoint presentation
- a visual display (this requires photographic evidence)
- a recorded lecture or presentation
- a podcast — one enhanced with graphics would give more detail
- a short video presentation
- a web page

Task guidance

To start with, you need to research the local provision and opportunities at grass roots and first level elite selection (this means a school or college first team) for participation in one chosen activity. Your project needs to reflect the school, college, club and area provisions in terms of facilities, organisations, competitions and performer development in the three roles of performer, leader and official.

Questions to consider when starting your research could include:
- How are my local facilities funded?
- Who provides and organises my chosen activity at the foundation level locally?
- Who provides and organises my activity at the participation and competitive levels locally?
- Are there any examples of elite provision locally?
- Which agencies provide funding and support to the sports clubs and facilities in my local area?
- What are the issues that face participants when considering regional differences in provision?
- What is the cost of taking part in my chosen activity locally (this could include cost of hiring the facility or court, annual and weekly membership of a sports club etc.)?
- How do these fees compare nationally?

How many of these questions can you answer already? You now need to plan how you can discover the information you require to answer the rest of them.

Resources for your local sports project
- **Internet** — the internet is a useful starting point. Your local council website might contain information on the type of activities played locally; it might also have links

directly to other local organisations' websites. Do any of your local sports clubs have their own websites? (These are usually fairly basic but they might give details of membership costs and times of training.) Sport England's website (**www.sportengland.org**) contains data on sport in your local area but may not mention specific sports in detail.

- **Local library** — local libraries often have a section dedicated to local activities and information on groups and clubs; staff may be able to direct you to surveys or reports that have been done on sport and recreation locally.
- **Local sports centres** — these are probably places where a lot of community sport is played. Look at notice boards — leagues and fixtures are often displayed, which will give you an insight into the numbers of teams and players involved. The sports centre may be able to give you links to local sports clubs. Ask for a copy of each centre's programme and look particularly at sessions that are provided for specific target groups. This will give you an idea of who is using the facilities. Price lists and/or a phone call to each centre's reception will give you an idea of the costs involved in playing your sport. Are there any private sector sports facilities locally, and how do these compare? For example, if you are studying football, are there any Powerleague or other private five-a-side centres local to you?
- **Local paper** — this should give you an overview of the number of local leagues and teams that play. Papers often feature specific sports on different days. Is there a weekend sports edition? (This would be useful for looking at grass-roots provision.) Most local papers have good websites where you can look at past issues — it may be worth searching for your sport. You may find that your local paper, like the national daily papers, focuses on a few sports.
- **Schools** — you need to include the provision for sport at both primary and secondary level in your presentation, so your school sports partnership is a good starting point. See if your school or college sports coordinator can give a presentation on what sports and schemes the partnership currently offers.
- **Local sports club** — if you play for a local sports club, finding information on things such as membership fees should be straightforward. If you don't, do you know a friend or relative who plays for a club? Check to see if the club has got a website. Many sports clubs have a joining handbook, which could also be a useful source of information.
- **Local council** — most local councils have a sports development unit, which should have a good overview of the provision for sports in the local area. Many also provide a brochure or web-based resource that lists all the sports facilities in the local area; this could be useful to cross-reference against your own sport.
- **County sports partnerships** — these should be able to provide you with a good overview of sport in your local area. Most have extensive websites and, if you are lucky, specific sections on individual sports.
- **National governing bodies** — NGBs may have information on sport locally and most NGB websites have a clubs directory so you can search for all the clubs in your local area. The key here is to identify the grass-roots schemes that your NGB runs; can you identify or find any of them in your local area?

- **National lottery** — the national lottery website (**www.national-lottery.co.uk**) lists all the awards given to individual sports and to local clubs and organisations.

What do I need to cover?

Local examples of provision at grass roots to first elite level of performance

This requires an overview of your chosen activity in the local area, to include numbers of people playing, the number of clubs, leagues and facilities available, and a description of the different levels within the performance pyramid.

Provision at local schools and colleges

You must provide an overview of your activity in the local schools and colleges, in which you need to chart the facilities and find out whether these are used by community groups and clubs as well.

Provision by at least one local sports club

Include a detailed description of the organisation, funding and sports provision. Provide facts such as how much it costs to join the club, where members train and play and how the funds required to run the club are raised. Where does the club fit into the sports performance pyramid? What external bodies have helped finance the club? Look for any link to the national lottery sports fund.

An overview of the facilities and opportunities available in the three key sectors

The three sectors are:

- the public sector — owned and run by local councils, to include state-run schools and colleges
- the private sector — owned and run by commercial companies, to include private schools or colleges in the area
- the voluntary sector — where the organisation is run by volunteers, i.e. people who give up their time free of charge, to include community groups and clubs

Schemes and programmes available in your activity

These will normally be national programmes developed by your sports governing body but delivered locally through schools, clubs and community facilities. Look for examples of mini versions of your sport that may be delivered by primary schools and junior clubs (examples include mini rugby, high five netball, kwik cricket). Some sports offer award schemes for young participants (examples include swimming or gymnastics awards and star:track athletics). You might also be able to research local examples aimed at other community groups. For instance, does your local sports facility run programmes for older participants (often called 'ageing well' sessions)?

Performer development for player, leader and official

You need to produce pathways of development for each of the roles, which might be best done through a series of diagrams. You might find the outline of the pathways on your sports national governing body website, but remember that you need to localise these pathways. Are all the opportunities available in your local area?

Provision and support for disabled participants in the local area

What are the opportunities for disabled people in your local area? Are there any specific clubs available or do existing clubs offer opportunities for participants with disability? How well do the local sports facilities cater for participants with disability? How does your area compare with the national picture?

Gender issues relating to the provision of the sport locally

Is your sport open to participants regardless of gender, or is there a gender bias? How does the local area compare with the national picture? Are any clubs or facilities in the local area specifically targeting gender issues?

> **Tip** Check out the Women's Sports Foundation website (**www.womenssports foundation.org**). Is there any reference to your sport?

Reference your work

You must reference your work fully. This means indicating the resources you have used and stating where you have used words, facts and diagrams from any external sources. As a rough guide, your assignment should be at least 90% your own words and work.

All references and sources you have used should be listed in a bibliography at the end of your assignment. Books should be referenced using the 'Harvard system', where the sequence is as follows: name of author, book title, year of publication and/or edition and publisher. Websites should be listed, along with a short description of what each site contains (don't include search engines). The external examiners will check the websites you have listed, so make sure that the details are correct. Don't forget to include any magazines and publications you have used. Finally, remember to mention any people who have helped you with the assignment, specifying their position and explaining in a few lines how they helped you.

Critique on your research

You should include some comments about your research and presentation of Task 2.2. How easy was it to find the information on your activity locally? What or who was the best source of information? If you were to repeat the task, what would you do differently? What do you think are the strengths and weaknesses of your presentation? You should link the study to one of the roles you are being assessed in for Task 2.1 (performer/leader/official), concentrating on the opportunities and pathways available to either a performer in your sport or a leader or official in your sport.

You should refer to your bibliography in your critique and make a judgement on how easy it was to find the information you required. When your assignment is ready, your teacher will ask you to complete an authentication statement asking you to confirm that the work you are submitting is your own.

How will I score marks on this assignment?

Your centre assessor and the external examiner will read through your assignment several times and then use a grid similar to the one below to give your project a mark out of 15. You can use this grid as a checklist for your own assignment. Although most of the content reads the same, there are key words to look for in each phrase — we have put these in bold to make them easier for you to identify.

Band	Description
Band 5 13–15 marks	The project demonstrates a **very high level** of knowledge and understanding of the local provision in the chosen physical activity. It has **fully explored** the provision, opportunities and resources available at grass-roots level and at the first level of elite representation. There is a **detailed overview** of the provision and opportunities available at school and/or college and clubs, and the wider provision and opportunities available through both public and private facilities and resources, including the part played by the voluntary sector. **Full reference** has been made to the various schemes open to participants, the funding of such provision and the additional agencies and bodies involved. **Detailed reference** has been made to the provision for disabled athletes and to any gender issues. There are **appropriate** critical comments on the findings. The project includes **significant** factual detail and contains an **extensive** bibliography. It contains reference to the development opportunities in at least one of the roles selected for Task 2.1.
Band 4 10–12 marks	The project demonstrates a **high level** of knowledge and understanding of the local provision in the chosen physical activity. It contains a **sound overview** of the provision, opportunities and resources available at grass-roots level and at the first level of elite representation. There is a **sound review** of the provision and opportunities available at school and/or college and clubs, and the wider provision and opportunities available through both public and private facilities and resources, including the part played by the voluntary sector, although there are **some omissions**. **Reference** has been made to the various schemes open to participants, the funding of such provision and the additional agencies and bodies involved. **Some reference** has been made to the provision and opportunities for disabled athletes and to any gender issues. There is **some** critical comment on the findings. The project includes **a range** of factual detail and contains an **appropriate** bibliography. In most areas it contains reference to the development opportunities in at least one of the roles selected for Task 2.1. *continued*

Band	Description
Band 3 7–9 marks	The project demonstrates a **good level** of knowledge and understanding of the local provision in the chosen physical activity. **An attempt** has been made to explore the provision, opportunities and resources available at grass-roots level and at the first level of elite representation, with some success. The project **has attempted** to establish the provision and opportunities available at school and/or college and clubs, and the wider provision and opportunities available through both public and private facilities and resources, including the part played by the voluntary sector, although there are **clear omissions**. **Some reference** has been made to the various schemes open to participants, the funding of such provision and the additional agencies and bodies involved. **Some reference** has been made to the provision and opportunities for disabled athletes and to any gender issues. There is **some** critical comment on the findings. The project contains a bibliography. **Limited reference** has been made to the development opportunities in at least one of the roles selected for Task 2.1.
Band 2 4–6 marks	The project demonstrates a **moderate level** of knowledge and understanding of the local provision in the chosen physical activity. **An attempt** has been made to explore the provision, opportunities and resources available at grass-roots level and at the first level of elite representation. The candidate **may have attempted** to establish the provision and opportunities available at school and/or college and clubs, and the wider provision and opportunities available through both public and private facilities and resources, including the part played by the voluntary sector, although there are **significant omissions**. **Limited reference** has been made to the various schemes open to participants, the funding of such provision and the additional agencies and bodies involved. **Little reference** has been made to the provision and opportunities for disabled athletes and to any gender issues. There are **simplistic** critical comments on the findings. The project **may not** contain an appropriate bibliography. There are **few factual** inclusions and **limited reference** to the development opportunities in at least one of the roles selected for Task 2.1.
Band 1 1–3 marks	The project demonstrates a **limited** level of knowledge and understanding of the local provision in the chosen physical activity. It has **largely failed** to explore the provision, opportunities and resources available at grass-roots level and at the first level of elite representation. The candidate has been **unable** to establish the provision and opportunities available at school and/or college and clubs, and the wider provision and *continued*

Band	Description
	opportunities available through both public and private facilities and resources, including the part played by the voluntary sector, and the task contains **significant omissions**.
	Scant reference has been made to the various schemes open to participants, the funding of such provision and the additional agencies and bodies involved.
	There is only a **simple** review or reference to the provisions and opportunities for disabled athletes and/or to any gender issues.
	There are **no**, or only **simplistic**, critical comments on the findings.
	The project **may not** contain an appropriate bibliography.
	Factual detail has been **omitted** and there is **no reference** to the development opportunities in at least one of the roles selected for Task 2.1.

Final checklist

Item required	Tick when completed
I have included details of local examples of sports provision at grass roots to first level of elite performance.	
I have included provision at local schools and colleges.	
I have included provision in at least one local sports club.	
I have included reference to facilities and opportunities in the following sectors: • public • private • voluntary	
I have mentioned the schemes and programmes available in my chosen physical activity.	
I have mentioned the agencies that support and fund the activity in my local area.	
I have explained the development pathways for the three roles: performer, leader and official.	
I have identified the provision and support for disabled participants in my local area.	
I have discussed gender issues relating to the provision of my activity locally.	
I have made critical comments about my research and presentation of Task 2.2.	
I have linked my study to one of the roles I am being assessed in for Task 2.1 (performer/leader/official).	
I have included a bibliography.	

Task 2.3: national study

Key points

- You need to select one role from performer, leader or official and give a detailed development pathway from initial elite selection (school/college first team) to national representation.
- You need to explain the support given to elite performers in your chosen physical activity.
- You need to describe the national governing body (NGB) provisions for your activity at the national level.

How will you be assessed?

There is no set format for Task 2.3, so you can present your work in a range of ways. You should choose a style that you are familiar with or that you think will best present the information you discover on your sport nationally.

Your presentation must be limited to 1,000 words if you are writing in continuous prose. Teacher assessors and moderators will discontinue marking once the prescribed word limit is reached.

Some examples of the type of format you could choose include:

- a brochure that illustrates your sport nationally
- a PowerPoint presentation
- a visual display (this requires photographic evidence)
- a recorded lecture or presentation
- a podcast — one enhanced with graphics would give more detail
- a short video presentation
- a web page

Task guidance

Task 2.3, the national study, builds on the work you have completed for Task 2.2, the local study. The focus of this task is to identify the elite pathways and national provision in one of your chosen roles from Task 2.1 (performer, leader or official). You need to track each of the levels of development from first elite level through to national representation in your sport. You also need to describe the support that is available to participants at each level. The phrase 'first elite level' refers to a stage equivalent to an educational establishment first team (i.e. school or college), but for some sports this may not be straightforward so you may need to discuss this with your teachers.

Questions to consider when starting your research could include:

- How are the national facilities for my chosen sport funded?
- Who is responsible for organising my sport at the national level? (You need to cover all the levels of the participation pyramid.)

- Who are the agencies providing funding and support to the sports clubs and facilities nationally?
- How are elite performers supported at the national level?
- What are the issues that face participants accessing all levels of my sport?

How many of these questions can you answer already? You now need to plan how you can discover the information you require to answer the rest of them.

Resources for your national sports project

- **Internet** — the internet is a useful starting point. However, you may not always find information regarding the national provision of your activity and your chosen role.
- **UKSIs/national sports centres** — these are facilities that are used by elite performers, leaders and officials for training and monitoring. Most have websites where you can research the services they offer. There should be one fairly close to you and it may be worth visiting it to see how it helps to prepare and support elite athletes at different stages of the elite pathway.
- **UK Sport** — this is the key national agency that manages elite sport. It has direct responsibility for most elite performers and supports athletes at the elite stages of development. The agency's website is definitely worth a visit — go to **www.uksport.gov.uk**.
- **Schools** — you need to include the role of schools and colleges in the first stage of talent identification and channelling talented performers into the appropriate pathways.
- **Local elite sports club** — which club plays at the highest level in your locality (it needs to be playing in a national level league)? Check to see if the club has a website. Find out when match day is and go along to have a look at the provision. You may also be able to make contact with someone who can give you more information on the work of the club.
- **National governing bodies** — NGBs should have information on the elite pathway and may also have separate sections for leaders and officials.
- **National lottery** — the national lottery website (**www.national-lottery.co.uk**) lists all the awards given to individual sports and to local clubs and organisations.
- **Additional agencies** — specialist organisations such as Sports Coach UK (**www.sportscoachuk.org**), Sports Leaders UK (**www.sportsleaders.org**) and the Women's Sports Foundation (**www.womenssportsfoundation.org**) have websites that offer good sources of information on how these bodies support elite sport in the UK.

What do I need to cover?

Structure and pathway

Having chosen your preferred role, you need to represent the stages of development from first elite level through to national representation — perhaps best illustrated in a pyramid diagram.

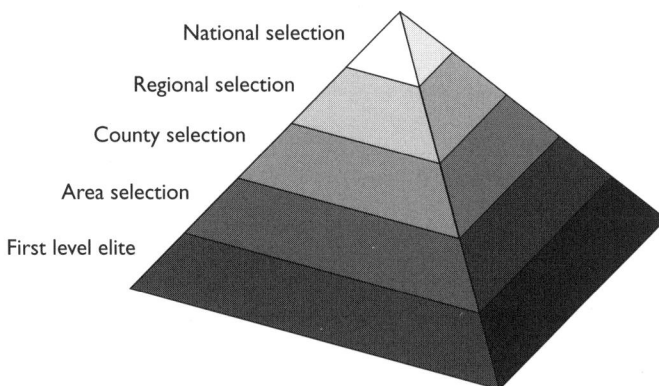

You should give a detailed description of each stage, and it is good practice to use a case study, that is, a named individual, so that you can explain fully the demands of each stage of development. Remember that for some sports there may be more than one pathway, so you may need to provide more than one diagram.

Role and function of sporting academies

Your first task is to research whether your activity supports elite participants through sports academies. Places at academies may be offered as part of the UK Sport's World Class Programme or, as in the case of football, they may be run at a club/local level. Academies tend to focus their work on developing young talent and preparing players for their transition into the national stage of the elite pathway.

Process of talent identification

How does your activity identify talent and select performers for each of the stages in the elite sports pathway? The national governing body websites are a good place to start, and personal experience from friends or acquaintances who have been through the selection process may also be a great source of information. Remember, there will be pathways for performers, leaders and officials.

Role played by schools and clubs, area and county sports associations

This section links to the three above. Schools and colleges tend to be involved with the first stage of the elite pathway. Look for schools and colleges that offer specific support programmes for elite performers — a couple of case studies could be used here. Some colleges are labelled as sports academies. Again, personal experience of the county level of the pathway may be the best source of information. Do you know anyone who has played your sport or coached/officiated at this level?

Role played by national governing bodies and professional structures

This section links into the elite pathways. How do NGBs support the pathways? (The NGB website is a good starting point.) Some activities offer apprenticeships for developing talent — these usually come under the Advanced Apprenticeship in Sports Excellence (AASE) model, which may be worth investigating for your own activity. Does your activity also offer fast-track programmes for young coaches or officials? For those activities that have a professional stage, there will be a players' association — examples include the Professional Footballers' Association (**www.givemefootball.com**) and the Professional Golfers' Association (**www.pga.info**). Check to see if your own activity has such a website and find out what support is offered to elite performers.

Schemes and funding open to participants

We have already touched on these in the section above. Most Olympic sports work within UK Sport's World Class Programme, which is supported by the national lottery. The UK Sport website gives details of elite sports funding (**www.uksport.gov.uk**). Some professional sports, such as cricket, offer a central contract scheme for the national level of the pathway. There are sports-specific programmes for leaders and officials, details of which can be found on your national governing body website. Sports Aid is a charity that supports young emerging talented performers — check out the website at **www.sportsaid.org.uk** to research links to your own activity.

Additional agencies and bodies involved in supporting the pathway

If you have chosen the performer pathway, you need to research the role that UK Sport plays in your activity. For the leader pathway, Sports Leaders UK (**www.sportsleaders.org**) and Sports Coach UK (**www.sportscoachuk.org**) need to be mentioned. It may be more difficult to find additional agencies that support officials, but check out the Central Council of Physical Recreation (CCPR) website at **www.ccpr.org.uk** and Sport England (**www.sportengland.org**).

Elite provision for disabled participants

For most sports, disabled athletes follow a parallel system within the UK Sport's World Class Programme. Your first check should be whether your activity is a Paralympic sport or whether the UK sends teams to other world disability sport competitions. Good links are the British Paralympic Association (**www.paralympics.org.uk**) and the English Federation of Disability Sport (**www.efds.net**).

Gender issues in elite provision

Does your activity offer elite opportunities to participants regardless of gender, or is there a gender bias? How does the UK compare with other nations? You may find that there are national teams for both genders but only the male teams get media coverage. The Women's Sports Foundation is a good starting point.

Reference your work

You must reference your work fully. This means indicating the resources you have used and stating where you have used words, facts and diagrams from any external sources. As a rough guide, your assignment should be at least 90% your own words and work.

All references and sources you have used should be listed in a bibliography at the end of your assignment. Books should be referenced using the 'Harvard system', where the sequence is as follows: name of author, book title, year of publication and/or edition and publisher. Websites should be listed with a short description of what each site contains (don't include search engines). The external examiners will check the websites you have listed, so make sure the details are correct. Don't forget to include any magazines and publications you have used. Finally, remember to mention any people who have helped you with the assignment, specifying their position and explaining in a few lines how they helped you.

Critique on your research

Include some comments about your research and presentation of Task 2.3. How easy was it to find the information on your activity nationally? What or who was the best source of information? If you were to repeat the task, what would you do differently? What do you think are the strengths and weaknesses of your presentation? You should link the study to one of the roles you are being assessed in for Task 2.1 (performer/ leader/official). Where are you on the performance pathway you presented at the start of the task?

You should refer to your bibliography in your critique and make a judgement on how easy it was to find the information you required. When your assignment is ready, your teacher will ask you to complete an authentication statement asking you to confirm that the work you are submitting is your own.

How will I score marks on this assignment?

Your centre assessor and the external examiner will read through the assignment several times and then use a grid similar to the one below to give your project a mark out of 15. You can use this grid as a checklist for your own assignment. Although most of the content reads the same, there are key words to look for in each phrase — we have put these in bold to make them easier for you to identify.

Mark band	Description
Band 5 13–15 marks	The project demonstrates a **very high level** of knowledge and understanding of the national provision in the chosen physical activity. It includes a **detailed overview** of the structures, pathways and provisions for a chosen role. There is a **good level of detail** regarding the role and functions of sporting academies, the process of talent identification, the role played by schools, clubs, area and county associations and the part played by NGBs and professional structures. **Full reference** is made to the various schemes open to participants, the funding of such provisions and the additional agencies and bodies involved. It contains a **detailed review** of the elite provisions and opportunities for disabled athletes in the activity and/or participation role, and reference is made to any gender issues. There are **appropriate** critical comments on the findings and **significant factual detail** is included. The project contains an **extensive** bibliography.

continued

Mark band	Description
Band 4 10–12 marks	The project demonstrates a **high level** of knowledge and understanding of the national provision in the chosen physical activity. It includes a **sound overview** of the structures, pathways and provisions for a chosen role, although there may be **some omissions**. **An attempt** has been made to establish the role and functions of sporting academies and the process of talent identification. There is a **sound description** of the role played by schools, clubs, area and county associations, NGBs and professional structures. **Some reference** is made to the various schemes open to participants, the funding of such provisions and the additional agencies and bodies involved. It contains **mention** of the elite provisions and opportunities for disabled athletes in the activity and/or participation role, and reference is made to any gender issues. There are **some** critical comments on the findings and a **range of factual detail** is included. The project contains an **appropriate** bibliography.
Band 3 7–9 marks	The project demonstrates a **good level** of knowledge and understanding of the national provision in the chosen physical activity. It includes **an attempt** to explore the structures, pathways and provisions for a chosen role, although there are **clear omissions**. There is some **description** of the role and functions of sporting academies and the process of talent identification, along with **some information** on the role played by schools, clubs, area and county associations, NGBs and professional structures. **Some reference** is made to the various schemes open to participants, the funding of such provisions and the additional agencies and bodies involved. It contains **limited mention** of the elite provisions and opportunities for disabled athletes and/or gender issues. There are **some** critical comments on the findings and **some factual detail** is included. The project contains a bibliography.
Band 2 4–6 marks	The project demonstrates a **moderate level** of knowledge and understanding of the national provision in the chosen physical activity. It includes **limited description** of the structures, pathways and provisions for the chosen role. There is **an attempt** to establish the role and functions of sporting academies and the process of talent identification. However, there is **limited or no detailed information** pertaining to the role played by schools, clubs, area and county associations, NGBs and professional structures. **Limited reference** is made to the various schemes open to participants, the funding of such provisions and the additional agencies and bodies involved. It contains **limited mention** of the elite provisions and opportunities for disabled athletes in the activity and/or participation role, and only **limited** reference to any gender issues. There are **simplistic** critical comments on the findings and **few factual details**. The project **may not** contain an appropriate bibliography.

continued

Mark band	Description
Band 1 1–3 marks	The project shows only a **limited level** of knowledge and understanding of the national provision in the chosen physical activity. It **fails** to explore the structures, pathways and provisions for a chosen role and there are **significant omissions**. There may be **some attempt** to establish the role and functions of sporting academies and the process of talent identification. However, the task **fails** to contain detailed information pertaining to the role played by schools, clubs, area and county associations, NGBs and professional structures. **Scant reference** is made to the various schemes open to participants, the funding of such provisions and the additional agencies and bodies involved. It contains only **brief mention** of the elite provisions and opportunities for disabled athletes in the activity and/or participation role, and makes no reference to any gender issues. There are **no critical comments** on the findings and **factual details have been omitted**. The project may not contain an appropriate bibliography.

Final checklist

Item required	Tick when completed
I have included the structure and pathway for elite development for my chosen role in my chosen activity from first elite level to national representation.	
I have included the role and function of sporting academies.	
I have described the process of talent identification in my chosen activity.	
I have described the role played by schools and clubs, area and county sports associations.	
I have described the role played by national governing bodies and professional structures.	
I have mentioned the schemes and funding open to participants.	
I have identified the additional agencies and bodies involved in supporting the pathway.	
I have identified the provision and support for disabled participants.	
I have discussed gender issues relating to the provision of my activity nationally.	
I have made critical comments about my research and presentation of Task 2.3.	
I have linked my study to one of the roles I am being assessed in for Task 2.1 (performer/leader/official).	
I have included a bibliography.	

Task 2.4: performance analysis

Key points

The final task in Unit 2 requires you to analyse performance. The performance that you analyse must be related to one of the two roles that you were assessed in for Task 2.1. Consequently you will be analysing the performance of a performer, a leader or an official. Your analysis will be assessed and marked out of 30.

By developing a critical analysis through independent research, you should build knowledge of the expectations of your chosen role and be able to recognise the strengths and weaknesses in your own performance. This should allow you to improve your own performance.

In this section we explain what analysis of performance actually means, why we would wish to analyse performance and how we should go about it.

How will you be assessed?

You need to complete five assignments that cover the following areas:
- a technical analysis of four core skills in a chosen activity
- a tactical analysis including game plans and pathways for competitive success in a variety of competition contexts
- three notational exercises on teams, individuals or techniques
- a training analysis on the sport-specific demands and the competitive require-ments for individuals and/or teams
- an analysis of your own and others' strengths and weaknesses

Key terms

Technical analysis — this involves identifying the core skills and breaking them down into their four constituent parts: technical, tactical, physiological and mechanical.

Notational exercise — an exercise in which you record the activity of a specific performer, team or technique during a period of play.

Training analysis — this involves identifying the training requirements of the role you have chosen; you need to cover physiological, mechanical and tactical elements.

Assignment 1: technical analysis

You need to identify four skills required in your chosen role in your chosen activity. These skills then need to be broken down into their four constituent parts: technical, tactical, physiological and mechanical. You need to present a visual record of the four skills you have identified. This can be done through video footage or photographs of yourself and, to allow comparison, of an elite performer. You may find technical journals and websites useful in breaking down each skill into the phases of perform-ance. The BBC Sport Academy website (**www.bbc.net.uk/sportacademy**) may prove valuable here.

For example, if you choose the role of an official, you could select the four skills of positioning, verbal communication, physical communication and physiological requirements. If you choose the role of leader, you could select the skills of verbal and non-verbal communication, demonstrating skills and coaching styles that are appropriate to the task. If you choose the role of performer, you need to demonstrate your understanding of the performance to be carried out (perfect model) and the ability to observe, compare, plan and communicate.

Assignment 2: tactical analysis

This analysis can be of a team or an individual performance (of a performer, leader or official). Possible subjects for study include critical comparisons of the effectiveness of different formations used in sports such as rugby, football or basketball; or comparing set plays such as a centre pass in netball, or short corners in hockey. In individual sports such as athletics, you could look at the different approaches athletes use in heats and/or qualification rounds compared with those they apply in finals.

Assignment 3: notational exercise

You need to carry out three notational or computer analyses for one of your chosen roles. The analyses can be based on a whole team, a positional unit (such as the back four in football or the pack in rugby) or an individual performance. Although it is possible to use a range of formats, it is best to stick to the same format for all three analyses so that comparisons can be made.

Notational analysis involves using notes, symbols or figures to record events, skills and scores in a sports competition. It can be done 'live' (i.e. while actually watching the sport) or using video material after the event. It may be better to practise using video clips to start with. Normally, a tally of events is taken during the action, and then after the game totals can be calculated and analysis done. Below is an example of a notation sheet for a rugby player. This could be adapted for a sport of your choice.

Match analysis — game sheet					
Player:			Position:		
Event	First half		Second half		
	Tally	Total	Tally	Total	Totals
Passes made					
Passes received					
Tackles made					
Tackles successful					
Runs made					
Tackles broken					
Off loads					
Ball dropped					
Kicks received					
Kicks made					

Assignment 4: training analysis

You need to identify, and create a presentation on, the training requirements of the role you have chosen, covering physiological, mechanical and tactical elements. You can use your own experiences or those of others, including elite performers, in order to highlight the specific requirements. There are key links to Unit 1 and you may want to review your notes and lessons from that unit.

Assignment 5: strengths and weaknesses

This involves carrying out an analysis of your own and, if appropriate, other performers' strengths and weaknesses during performance. You need to make full use of the knowledge and understanding you have gained through the other four analysis assignments. You can present the strengths and weaknesses in a written, digital or photographic format, for example:

	Strengths	Weaknesses
Performer	Good, consistent application of skills.	Poor decision-making, i.e. performed the skill accurately but chose the wrong skill.
Leader	Generally a very good motivator, able to get the performers aroused to optimum level.	Relatively poor tactician. Unable to adapt to strengths of opponents.
Official	Is able to keep up with play and consistently applies the roles well.	Makes decisions a little too quickly. Could allow the situation to develop a little first.

Why analyse performance?

There are several reasons why you might want to analyse your performance or that of another athlete or team. By analysing performance you can understand exactly what is happening. Only when you understand what is happening can you begin to work out why. Then you can:

- correct mistakes that you have made
- repeat your successes
- understand your opponents' tactics and strategies
- employ the most appropriate tactics against your opponents

How do you analyse performance?

It sounds simple but analysing performance properly is not easy unless you know what you are trying to do. For example, during his tenure as England football manager, Kevin Keegan was asked at half time in a game against Germany (which England was losing) what was going wrong. He replied that the players were not passing the ball very well. He was then asked what he had told the players to help them. He looked at the interviewer incredulously before replying, 'I've told them to pass it better this half.' In this case, Keegan did not know how to analyse performance. No player would pass the ball badly on purpose, so Keegan's 'helpful' comments would have been totally useless to the players. They needed to know *why* they were not passing the ball well enough. Were they taking too much time on the ball, or taking too many touches? Were team-mates not creating effective angles to be passed to? Was the opposition closing them down too quickly? By not identifying *why* things were not working, Keegan was unable to plan effectively how to change things and so as a coach he was of no significant help to his team.

Being able to analyse performance properly enables you to plan effectively and appropriately. To analyse performance, you must first know what you are looking for. Once that is clear, you need to be able to compare what you have seen with what you wanted to see, identify the differences, and communicate the need to change in a way that facilitates the changes desired and so creates what you wanted in the first place.

What you are looking for is the 'perfect model' — what the perfect execution of the skill would look like. You therefore need to know the fine details of the skill in order to understand what has gone wrong.

When you watch a skill, what do you actually see? Is it the end product or the process that produces the product? Observing a skill in detail is a skill in itself and one that you need to develop. It certainly becomes easier with practice. It is easier to see what is really going on when you know more about the skill itself. So explaining the perfect model in detail will help you to see more clearly what is actually happening.

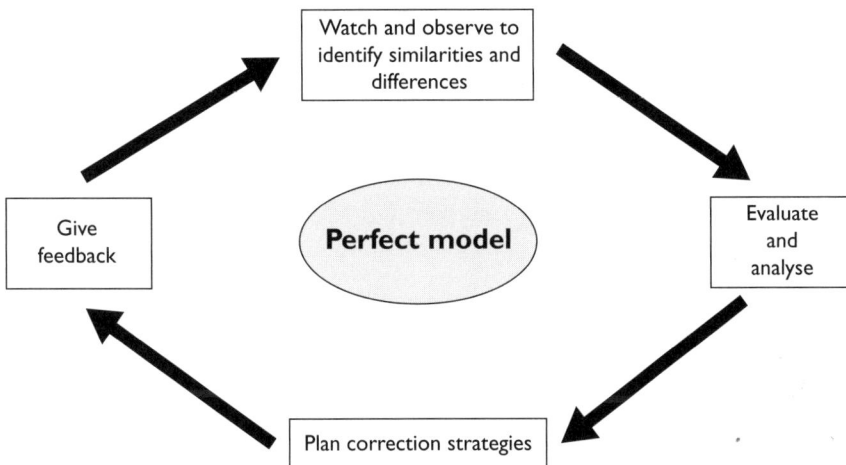

There are often several different ways of performing the same skill. Watch two golfers teeing off from the same tee in a golf match — their swings can look completely different from one another. Because of this, when we watch a skill or performance we must first work out the desired outcome. This is called the evaluation and it involves applying value to the outcome (see p. 52). Next you need to make judgements to support your evaluation. These usually relate to the perfect model and highlight where there is a difference between the two.

Next comes the tricky bit. You know what's wrong, now you have to fix it. You need to transform what you saw into what you want to see. How you do this depends very much on the skill and level of experience of the performer, the degree of error, the time scale, and the equipment and resources available to you.

The way in which you communicate what you saw and your suggested follow-up instructions is critical to the eventual success, or lack of it, for the performer.

And then the whole process begins again, to be repeated until the result is perfect.

In summary:
- You need to be able to identify similarities and differences between what is happening and what should be happening.
- To do that, you must know what the performance *should* be like. This is known as the **perfect model**.
- Then you need to **evaluate** the real performance against the perfect model.
- Next you must **analyse** your evaluation so that you are aware of what needs to be improved.
- You then need to plan and implement the appropriate changes to bring the real performance in line with the perfect model.

The perfect model

Before you can analyse a performance, you need to know what it should look like — this is referred to as the perfect model. The perfect model needs to be broken down into components to allow a detailed and thorough understanding. This also enables weaknesses to be more accurately pinpointed. One way is to break it down into chrono-logical order or a sequence of events. This would suit a discrete skill, such as a shot put, which has a short time span and a clearly defined beginning and end. For skills that have no clearly distinguishable starting and finishing points — continuous skills, such as a swimming stroke or the leg action in cycling — it may be easier to look at body movements and efficiency.

Chronological breakdown

To analyse a skill using this method, the skill should be broken down into stages to make it easier to understand. The four stages are:
- the **starting position** — this is the perfect position before the movement or skill begins
- the **transitional phase** — all the movements that are needed to get from the starting position to the point of execution
- **execution** — this is the actual skill
- **recovery** — the movements that are necessary to complete the skill while remaining in control

This type of breakdown lends itself well to detailed analysis. Once you have identi-fied the correct position for each stage and understood why each position is neces-sary or beneficial to the performance, you are more likely to understand what might be affecting the performance of a specific performer. Going through this order of events also makes it easier to analyse the performance. Often you will find that a poor starting position or transitional phase is causing the problems.

The table below shows an example of the stages in the hop of a shot put perfect model.

Physical position and efficiency of movement

Not all skills can be broken down into this sequence of events however. The front crawl stroke, or indeed any swimming stroke, the cycling action or running are all sporting examples of continuous skills that would be difficult to break down effectively as described above. For these types of skill it is easier to look at the movement in terms of:

- the arm action
- the leg action
- the head carriage/position
- the body position
- total body efficiency

In the same way as starting position and transition are often the causes of poor performance for discrete skills, so too is body position here. Getting the correct physical balance is often the key, because without it the performer will be compensating throughout the movement.

Chronological breakdown of the stages in the hop phase of a shot put

Stage	Description	How is it achieved	Why?
Starting position	• Stand at the back of the circle • Face the opposite direction to that in which you are going to throw • Stand on your throwing leg in a 'T' position, with a slight bend in the leg	• Move to the back of the circle • Stand with your back to the throwing area • Balance on your throwing leg with your non-throwing arm out to your side and your non-throwing leg behind you	• To use the distance to get more speed • To get extra speed and propulsion just before release as you twist around • For balance
Transition	• Sink down on your throwing leg • Push off quickly upwards and backwards • Upon landing approximately half way across the circle, again sink down on the throwing leg • Extend your non-throwing leg out behind you and place the foot on the ground	• Relax the quadriceps, allowing gravity to pull your body down. Ensure that your back remains relatively straight • Contract the quadriceps muscle, powerfully straightening the leg and bringing the body back to an upright position • As before • Contract the quadriceps of the non-throwing leg, extending it out towards the direction of the throw, placing the foot on the ground	• To incorporate the body's biggest and most powerful muscles (hamstring, quadriceps and gluteals), thus getting greater distance on the throw • See above • By hopping you incorporate the principle of plyometrics and get a more powerful contraction next time • For balance as you pivot and to incorporate the muscles from that leg too *continued*

Stage	Description	How is it achieved	Why?
Execution	● Pivot around the non-throwing leg, twisting at the waist as late as possible	● Rotate your body at the waist in the direction of the throwing area	● To get more power/speed just before release
	● At the same time, jump upwards from both the throwing leg and the non-throwing leg	● Contract the quadriceps and the gastrocnemius muscles, powerfully straightening the leg and bringing the body back to an upright position as you jump upwards	● To incorporate the body's biggest and most powerful muscles (hamstring, quadriceps and gluteals), thus getting greater distance on the throw, and consequently more speed, height and distance
	● At the same time extend the throwing arm, pushing the shot out at 45° from between horizontal and vertical	● Contract both the deltoid and triceps muscles of the throwing arm, extending the arm at 45°	● To push the shot out, gaining the optimum height for the maximum distance
	● Exhale aggressively	● Blow out all the air from your lungs as quickly as possible	● As it is an explosive event, the correct breathing technique is to exhale at the point of greatest exertion to obtain greatest power of contraction
Recovery	● Land facing the throwing area on the non-throwing leg, within the circle	● Pivot and jump during the first two phases of the execution stage	● To regain your balance while ensuring that you do not step out of the circle
	● Exit the circle from the back	● Walk out of the back of the circle after the throw	● To ensure that your throw is not disqualified

Evaluation stage

Before you begin to analyse, you must first know what the end product should be. We have discussed what it might look like, in terms of the perfect model, and this should shape your analysis. However, unless it is an aesthetic event, our preconceived notions of what the skill should look like must not dictate. A skill in sport is performed to achieve an end result and the end result must, to a large extent, be the determining factor of whether it is successful or not. For example, using the breakdown of sprinting as described above (i.e. the arm action, leg action, head carriage/position, body position, total body efficiency) and the specification marking criteria, how would you rate Michael Johnson, the retired American sprinter? It certainly would not be a top score because his body is far too upright, his knee lift is too low and his stride is too short.

But Michael Johnson was a world-class sprinter, who still holds world records in the 200 metres, 300 metres, 400 metres and 200 metres relay. He won five Olympic gold medals and was crowned world champion nine times. In 1996 he became the only male sprint athlete in history to win both the 200 metres and 400 metres events at the same Olympics, and the only man to successfully defend his title in the 400 metres at a Summer Olympics competition.

Consequently we must *evaluate* the performance before we analyse it and this must lead the discussion. If the result of the skill or performance is below what was hoped for, we can analyse why. If Michael Johnson was not running quickly, we could begin to look for reasons why that might be so. But since he was quick — very quick — we should evaluate his performance as being successful.

When evaluating, look for an objective against which to form your judgement. The penalty kick was successful because...it was a goal. The shot put was good because... it was a personal best. The front crawl stroke looks horrible but...he always wins the races. Regardless of how it looked (and as long as it was legal), the important question is — was it successful?

However, the opposite can also be true. A slightly built schoolgirl may have a textbook technique for the shot-put event but only manage to throw a distance of 5 metres. The evaluation of the throw would have to conclude that it was a poor throw. The analysis, however, might well reveal that all stages were a mirror image of the perfect model; it was a lack of power that resulted in the distance being poor.

Factors that affect performance

Many different factors affect performance, some of which have already been discussed. They can be categorised into four areas: physiological, psychological, technical and tactical.

Physiological

- Was the performance adversely affected by the level of fitness of the performer?
- Was the athlete injured, or not fully recovered from a previous injury?
- Was the athlete aware of all the components of fitness required for competition at the specific level and had he/she trained appropriately?
- Had the athlete warmed up appropriately and prepared sufficiently well for the conditions?

An example of an elite athlete failing as a result, arguably, of not preparing properly was when world champion Paula Radcliffe was forced to drop out of the Olympic marathon at the Athens 2004 Games. She refused to blame the hot Athens weather for her demise, but admitted: 'I felt there was nothing in my legs.' Many athletics experts suggested that she had not acclimatised to the local conditions, arriving in Athens only 3 days before the race.

Psychological

To many people, correct psychological preparation is just as important as physiological preparation.

- Athletes need to be highly motivated to train with the dedication needed to become fully fit and fully prepared.
- They need to be at the optimum level of arousal to perform to the best of their ability.
- They must focus on the task that they have to perform and give it their full attention, not allowing other people or events to distract them.
- They must have confidence in their own ability.
- They need to visualise success, but also, in many cases, failure so as to avoid experiencing it.

Choking is the inability to perform to an athlete's optimum performance — the sudden impairment or failure of sports performance due to anxiety. The harder one tries, the worse the performance. This is most likely caused by excessive self-consciousness and concern about the mechanics of skill execution. Famous examples include Ian Woosnam in golf and footballers failing in penalty shoot-outs. An athlete's potential for choking depends on both the athlete and the situation. Choking usually occurs when an athlete is overtly concerned about what others (team-mates, coaches, audience) think about their performance. Strategies to prevent choking include:

- setting one's own achievable goals
- using imagery prior to competition to review strategy and technique and create a sense of confidence
- using positive talk both in preparation and competition
- practising relaxation exercises
- using music prior to competition to help maintain focus by controlling negative thoughts

Technical

This refers to the ability of the performer to execute the required skills consistently to the highest level. It is the area that focuses on the attempted replication of the perfect model of a given skill or sporting movement. Biomechanical efficiency and analysis are significant here, as trajectory and efficiency can play a huge part in defining success or failure.

Equipment and clothing may be seen as an essential factor, as it can be what makes the difference between losing and winning. For example, in February 2008, Speedo launched its new revolutionary swimsuit, the LZR Racer. By April 2008, swimmers wearing the new suit had set 35 new world records, which led to questions being asked about the validity of the suit. One journalist called it 'doping on a hangar', while other swimsuit manufacturers asked the International Swimming Federation (FINA) to investigate the legality of the suit. Speedo designed the new suit in conjunction with NASA and the AIS. It has a tighter, corset-like mid-section, which is said to reduce fatigue at the end of a race. The suit is seamless and uses a water-repellent material that reduces drag in the water. Analysis of the swimming times of those using the new suit suggests an improvement of 2% in performance. Speedo responded to the criticisms by stating that while it had spent millions researching the new suit, other manufacturers had been focused on developing suits to follow fashion trends.

Tactical

Strategies and tactics play a huge part in most sports. In team games such as football, the number of tactics that can be used are almost endless and are equally endlessly debated — whether to play a 4–4–2 or a 5–3–2, whether to play an offside trap or to sit deep etc.

In individual sports such as athletics and swimming, tactics would be involved in a performer's race strategy: how he/she is going to run the race, what pace he/she will use at different stages and how to counter the strategies of other competitors. In racket sports, tactics might include when to play a baseline game or a serve-and-volley game in tennis.

Observational skills

Watching and really seeing what you are watching are skills that develop as you begin to practise carrying out proper analysis. Most people have an opinion on what should be done in order to change the direction of a sporting scenario. However, that opinion is often based on what they thought before the beginning of the event, rather than a result of what has happened so far. Consequently the suggested change may have little bearing, if any, on the outcome.

Watching an event with set targets, such as making a comparison against a perfect model, identifying strengths and weaknesses etc., will help you to focus on the event in more detail and, therefore, to see the process as well as the result.

Feedback

The manner in which you deliver feedback is essential if the analysis is to be effective. Your mode and style of delivery will depend heavily on the level of the performer and also on your knowledge of the athlete's personality. After all, different people respond very differently to particular styles of feedback.

A good place to start is for the performer to have a clear understanding of what he/she is aspiring to — i.e. what the perfect model looks like. You can provide this simply by telling the performer about your observations, or by demonstrating what you mean. However, it is perhaps most effective if you can show the performer a video, which can be slowed down or broken into parts.

> **Tip** Opinion is divided over whether common mistakes and pitfalls that need to be avoided should be shown. Some people believe it is helpful, as the performer can be made aware of what not to do. However, many experts now think that showing what should not be done could result in a subconscious adoption by the performer and may actually become the learned response.

The next step, which naturally follows on from this, is to identify how the performer's execution of the skill differs from the perfect model. This can be done through description, but you must remember that the majority of performers, having seen an example of the perfect model, will believe that their attempt looks exactly as it should. A more effective strategy, therefore, is to video the performer so that he/she can see clearly the difference between the two.

Once the weaknesses have been identified and understood, the performer needs help to move forward and adopt new techniques. With an elite performer, this might be done by explaining what needs to happen, with the use of appropriate technical language. At the lower end of the performance pyramid, performers will rely much more heavily on learning strategies and practices that have been created specifically to help foster the learning of the new skill. The simpler these are, the better the chance of success.

For example, when analysing a novice tennis player attempting to serve, it was noticed that the toss of the ball was slightly behind his head. The player had adapted to this and was consistently able to hit the ball into the appropriate service box. However, his opponents found it relatively easy to play a winning shot off what was supposed to be the server's advantage.

The analyser identified that because the toss was backwards rather than forwards, the player was hitting off the front foot rather than the back foot. This in turn resulted in a major loss of power. More importantly, it meant that the server was still on his back foot once the serve was made, leaving a lot of space for a simple cross-court return to be a winning shot.

The analyser gave the player a detailed breakdown of what his service looked like and what he needed to correct. All this was accurately explained using relevant technical language. However, the language was accurate but not appropriate; it was too advanced for the performer, who did not fully understand. The explanation was also too long to be effective — the performer thought that he was executing the shot as described. Consequently he listened, nodded and then performed the service exactly as before.

The analyser had watched the performance well, evaluated correctly and analysed effectively and in great detail. However, the value of all of this was lost because of inappropriate feedback.

An alternative style of feedback was tried. The tennis player was told to serve as normal, but that he would score a point if, after serving, he was able to run forward and touch the net before the return came back. No emphasis was placed on technicalities or on the service at all; indeed the player was told to serve as normal. The result was significant. In an attempt to get to the net quickly, the server naturally threw the ball forwards rather than backwards. The 'game' was soon adapted to telling the server to serve and then run forwards, playing the return if it came into his vicinity.

By adopting the latter style of feedback, the analyser was able to help the player adapt his technique effectively. Once this had been done, an explanation could be offered that identified why throwing the ball forwards was more effective.

Case study

Analysing the performance of an official

You will find that there is a lot more information available on observing and analysing the performance of a player, but it is easy to translate this material into methods and systems for viewing the performance of an official.

When you are preparing to watch and analyse the performance of an official, you need to choose the most appropriate methods of doing so. You need to identify:

- the strengths and weaknesses of the performance
- the relationship with other officials, players and coaches
- use of signals and effectiveness of communication
- decision-making and application of rules
- control of the game and any situations within it

Some sports offer assessor checklists on their websites. You could download these and use them to help you to create a version for use in your assessment. Remember that you may need to adapt these guidelines to suit the level of official you are analysing.

Bear in mind that officials will have their own style; this should not affect their interpretation of the rules, but it may mean that they deal with situations in different ways. The key, when analysing performance, is that the official shows consistency. Does he/she look comfortable with the chosen style and how do the players react to it?

Remember that you should be looking at both verbal and non-verbal communication, so judge the official when he/she makes verbal calls and also check that he/she is giving clear, correct signals. Also consider the emphasis given to calls; good officials are not as forceful on obvious calls, but show more decisiveness on close calls to reinforce their authority. If there are close calls, is a strong, clear voice used and are clear signals given? Effective communication also involves working with fellow officials, so check on the communication between them — again this should include verbal and non-verbal communication.

Blowing the whistle may appear to be a simple task but it is worth considering the different tones a whistle can give.

Improving the performance of an official
Most sports governing bodies have well-structured development pathways for referees and officials. It is a good idea to work out where the official you are analysing is on this pathway at present and try to discover what the next level might be in terms of progression. In order for an official to move up a level, it is usually necessary for him/her to undertake further training and some form of assessment. You need to identify what exactly is required for your specific case study and attempt to suggest where the official could attend a course or required training.

Improving fitness is a requirement for the higher levels of officiating, so it is useful to include an assessment of your chosen official's current fitness and suggestions for both targets and training plans that would enable him/her to meet the increased fitness demands.

Tip Key areas that you could consider when planning how to improve the performance of an official could include:
- practice
- training
- further qualifications
- self-analysis

- buddy systems (working with another official or more so that you can share advice and experiences)

There is a wide range of methods and programmes, examples of which are listed below, that you could consider when drawing up a development plan for a sports official you have worked with. The value of these depends both on the official you are working with and the specific sport.

- **Referee courses and retraining** — most governing bodies offer a pathway of progressive qualifications. The higher the level of qualification, the longer the courses are and the greater the demands on the official.
- **Websites** — there are a number of websites dedicated to officials in sport, which may offer ideas and techniques that you could apply to your official. Examples include **www.naso.org**, **www.referee.com** and **www.sportsofficialsuk.com**.
- **Special clinics** — local and regional associations often run clinics and workshops where officials can share ideas and discuss rules and regulations, and top-level officials are frequently invited to lead the sessions. Try to find out if your sport has local forums for sports officials.
- **Publications** — most governing bodies produce handbooks and guidelines for officials, which may be available as PDF downloads on websites. For more popular sports, such as football and tennis, there may be independent texts and handbooks, such as *An Introduction to Sports Officiating* by David Pegg (Coachwise Ltd, 2005), *Calling at Play: A Beginner's Guide to Amateur Sports Officiating* by Edward Dolan (Atheneum, 1981) and *Modern Sports Officiating: A Practical Guide* by Richard Clegg and William Thompson (Brown, 1989). As a minimum, make sure your official has up-to-date copies of the sports rules and regulations.
- **Officiating at local tournaments** — although it is hard work, having to referee a lot of short games played close together provides invaluable experience. It also creates the opportunity to watch and meet other officials.
- **Games** — refereeing or watching as many games as possible is the best way to develop knowledge and technique. Try to persuade your official to step up to officiate in adult or more senior games.
- **Assessors** — formal assessments are part of almost any governing body development pathway. They give valuable feedback and often contain specific areas for improvement. Assessors can be sounding boards too, and valuable for bouncing ideas and thoughts off.

Reference your work

You must reference your work fully. This means indicating the resources you have used and stating where you have used words, facts and diagrams from any external source. As a rough guide, your assignment should be at least 90% your own words and work.

All references and sources you have used should be listed in a bibliography at the end of your assignment. Books should be referenced using the 'Harvard system', where the sequence is as follows: name of author, book title, year of publication and/or edition and publisher. Websites should be listed with a short description of what each site contains (don't include search engines). The external examiners will check the websites you have listed, so make sure the details are correct. Don't forget to include any magazines and publications you have used. Finally, remember to mention any people who have helped you with the assignment, specifying their position and explaining in a few lines how they helped you.

When your assignment is ready, your teacher will ask you to complete an authentication statement asking you to confirm that the work you are submitting is your own.

How will I score marks on this project?

Your centre assessor and the external examiner will read through the assignment several times and then use a grid similar to the one below to give your analysis project a mark out of 30. You can use this grid as a checklist for your own assignment. Although most of the content reads the same, there are key words to look for in each phrase — we have put these in bold to make them easier for you to identify.

Each assignment has a total mark of 6. Your teachers will assess the evidence of the task undertaken in relation to the relevance and context of your chosen performance role and your standard or level of participation.

Mark band	Description
Band 5 25–30 marks	The task contains a **very high standard** of analysis that demonstrates a significant level of knowledge and understanding of the chosen role.
	There is **clear** technical accuracy and depth, and an **extensive range** of information.
	The task contains **varied and appropriate** presentation formats.
	The task offers a **full and extensive** application to performance of the specified role.
	The student has **fully completed** all analysis tasks linked to raising and developing his/her own and others' practical performance.
	The task is **fully** referenced with an **extensive** bibliography.
Band 4 19–24 marks	The task contains a **very good standard** of analysis that demonstrates a clear knowledge and understanding of the chosen role.
	There is **acceptable** technical accuracy and depth, and the range of information is **very good**.
	The clarity and use of appropriate presentation formats are **acceptable**.
	The task shows and discusses **relevant** application to performance of the specified role. However, the student may still need a **little prompting** in more complex situations.
	The student has **completed all** analysis tasks linked to raising and developing his/her own practical performance and on occasions has been able to influence the performance of others.
	The task is **referenced** with an **appropriate** bibliography.

continued

Mark band	Description
Band 3 13–18 marks	The task contains a **good standard** of analysis that demonstrates a general understanding of the chosen role. There is **reasonable** technical accuracy and some depth, and the range of information is **good**. The presentation formats used are **basic** in design. The task contains some **relevant** application to performance of the specified role. However, the student needs **prompting** in more complex situations. Some analysis tasks are **incomplete**, so the links to raising the student's own practical performance and being able to influence the performance of others are **limited**. The task contains **basic** references and a bibliography.
Band 2 7–12 marks	The task contains a **moderate** standard of analysis that demonstrates a limited knowledge and understanding of the chosen role. There is **some** technical accuracy and only **limited** information. The presentation formats are **simplistic** in design. The task contains **occasional limited** application to performance of the specified role, and a **significant level of prompting** is needed in order to discuss more complex situations. Some analysis tasks are **incomplete**, so the links to raising the student's own practical performance and being able to influence the performance of others are **limited**. The task contains **limited** references and a **limited** bibliography.
Band 1 1–6 marks	The task contains a **limited standard** of analysis that demonstrates a very limited knowledge and understanding of the chosen role. There is **no real** technical accuracy and **limited** information. The presentation formats are **very simplistic** in design. The student is **unable** to show any application to his/her own performance. The analysis tasks, in most cases, are **incomplete**, and have only enabled the student to apply a **basic** link to his/her own practical performance, resulting in an inability to influence the performance of others. The task contains **few**, if any, references and a **limited** bibliography.

Final checklist

Item required	Tick when completed
I have completed an analysis of four core skills.	
I have included reference to technical, tactical, physiological and mechanical aspects of these skills.	
I have completed a tactical analysis.	
I have completed three notational exercises.	
I have completed a training analysis — specific personal demands within the team/role context.	
I have made reference to physiological, tactical and mechanical requirements in my training analysis.	
I have included an analysis of my own strengths and weaknesses.	
I have included a bibliography.